Pendulum Healing

A Beginner's 5-Step Quick Start Guide to Unlocking Spiritual Healing and Connecting with your Chakras, With an FAQ

FELICITY PAULMAN

Disclaimer

By reading this disclaimer, you are accepting the terms of the disclaimer in full. If you disagree with this disclaimer, please do not read the guide.

All of the content within this guide is provided for informational and educational purposes only, and should not be accepted as independent medical or other professional advice. The author is not a doctor, physician, nurse, mental health provider, or registered nutritionist/dietician. Therefore, using and reading this guide does not establish any form of a physician-patient relationship.

Always consult with a physician or another qualified health provider with any issues or questions you might have regarding any sort of medical condition. Do not ever disregard any qualified professional medical advice or delay seeking that advice because of anything you have read in this guide. The information in this guide is not intended to be any sort of medical advice and should not be used in lieu of any medical advice by a licensed and qualified medical professional.

The information in this guide has been compiled from a variety of known sources. However, the author cannot attest to or guarantee the accuracy of each source and thus should not be held liable for any errors or omissions.

Introduction

Pendulum healing is a type of alternative healing practice that utilizes a pendulum device to diagnose and treat illness. The premise behind this technique is that physical, emotional, or spiritual imbalances in the body can be detected using the pendulum as a sort of divination tool.

To use a pendulum, one simply places the point at the end of the string or chain onto their body in an area where they are experiencing pain or discomfort. The movement of the pendulum over their body helps to discern any imbalances in their physical, mental, or emotional health, allowing them to make changes that restore balance and promote healing.

Once imbalances are recognized, they can then be addressed and corrected through various techniques including relaxation exercises, lifestyle changes, or even by using stones, crystals, and other natural elements.

Although there is no scientific evidence to support the validity of pendulum healing, many practitioners have found it to be an effective way to promote overall well-being and balance in the body and mind. Ultimately, whether you choose to use pendulum healing as part of your wellness routine is up to you. But before you dismiss it out of hand, it may be worth giving this age-old technique a try to see if it helps give you the boost that you need.

This beginner's guide will be an interesting one as we will deep-dive into each of the following subtopics:

- What is a pendulum?
- How does the pendulum work?
- Uses of the pendulum.
- Different pendulum materials.
- The different shapes of the pendulum.
- How to find a pendulum?
- 5-step guide to get started in using a pendulum.

So, read on to learn more about this fascinating and versatile healing tool, how to use it, and how it may benefit you. Whether you are looking to improve your overall health or manage specific symptoms of an illness, a pendulum can be a powerful ally in your quest for self-healing and well-being. Let's dive in!.

Table of Contents

WHAT IS A PENDULUM?

Pendulums are simple yet effective tools for healing and divination. An ancient healing tool, the pendulum is a simple yet powerful instrument that has been used for centuries to promote physical, emotional, and spiritual health.

Consisting of a weighted object suspended from a thin chain or thread, the pendulum acts like a tiny magnet, creating "waves" and cycles in the corresponding energy field as it moves back and forth. These waves can be directed and focused to target specific areas within the body for healing purposes.

Moreover, by holding conscious intent, a practitioner can use the pendulum to address deep-seated issues that may be affecting their overall well-being. With careful practice and guidance, anyone can successfully use this gentle yet highly effective healing tool.

Many modern healthcare practitioners utilize pendulums as a way to connect with their patient's energy fields and facilitate healing and well-being. These lightweight tools work by stimulating movement in intuitive and unconscious parts of the brain, offering a unique approach to addressing physical or emotional issues.

However, its efficacy depends on several factors, including an individual's motivation and the skill of the person performing the healing. Because of these complexities, pendulums are often best suited for more experienced practitioners and those who are highly attuned to their own body's energetic systems. Yet for those who are able, pendulums can be useful for promoting physical and emotional well-being, helping to clear stuck energies, and promoting deep and lasting healing.

Ultimately, a pendulum is just one of many tools that can be used in holistic healing practices, but it remains a valuable asset for those committed to exploring the transformative power of this ancient practice.

HOW DOES THE PENDULUM WORK?

Pendulums are lightweight metal or crystal tools that can easily be held in the palm of your hand or suspended on a chain. When you use a pendulum, you essentially put it into motion using small physical movements of your body and then wait for it to respond.

The various motions that a pendulum can make are thought to correspond with different levels of energy within the body. For example, circular or wobbly movements might be used to activate the abdominal region, while back-and-forth motions may be ideal for opening up blocked chakras and balancing the energies in the upper part of the body.

In general, many healers find that using a pendulum can help them tune into their intuitive insights about where an imbalance is located and what type of treatment will best address that imbalance.

The direction in which the pendulum moves can also offer valuable indications of your subconscious thoughts and feelings. For example, if you want to know whether you should accept a particular job offer and the pendulum swings downward over "yes," this may indicate that the decision is a good one.

Alternatively, opposing directions could mean that other options should be explored further before making any decisions about the job offer. Likewise, specific counterclockwise circles may indicate hesitation or uncertainty, while clockwise circles could suggest excitement or enthusiasm about this particular opportunity.

The use of pendulums has been used for centuries as a means of answering questions and finding insight. Essentially, pendulums work by utilizing our innate intuition and tapping into certain subconscious energies.

When asking a question, or holding a pendulum over an area of interest, the pendulum will move in response to the energetic vibrations that are present. This can enable us to find answers to important questions regarding everything from health and relationships to work and travel plans.

Whether you are new to using pendulums or have been relying on them for years, there are many benefits to using this simple yet powerful technology. For instance, pendulums can be used at any time, without anyone else being present or knowing about it. They can also provide clarity in situations where we may be feeling confused or unsure about the best course of action.

USES OF PENDULUM

Pendulums are often thought of as tools for divination and dowsing, but they can be used for a wide variety of purposes. From gaining insights to clearing energetic blocks, pendulums are versatile tools that everyone should have in their toolkit. Let's take a look at some of the many ways you can use a pendulum.

Dowsing and scrying: Dowsing and scrying are popular methods for exploring one's subconscious and obtaining valuable insights into the world around us. However, these processes can be challenging and frustrating for those who are new to them. In particular, there is often a lot of trial and error involved as individuals try to figure out the right method or technique that works best for them. Fortunately, using a pendulum is an effective way to facilitate dowsing and scrying, making it an ideal choice for beginners.

Pendulums can be a valuable tool for gaining insight into all aspects of our lives. By tapping into the wisdom of our higher selves and the akashic records, they allow us to gain deeper clarity around important questions and situations. Whether we are trying to make career choices, navigate relationships, or resolve other key issues, a pendulum can offer valuable guidance. With practice, this powerful tool can help us to make wise decisions and find greater fulfillment in every area of our lives.

Connect with your chakras: Pendulums are tools commonly used to connect with our chakras. Each of us has seven major energy centers, or chakras, within our bodies, through which the universal life force flows. By using a pendulum, we can learn to recognize the different vibrations and energies associated with each of our chakras. This helps us to better tune in to the energies around us and tap into deeper states of meditation and healing.

Many people believe that the movement and direction of a pendulum are influenced by different chakra energies. For example, some believe that hanging the pendulum from the root chakra will produce downward movements when particularly associated energy is present in the environment. Likewise, people may use pendulums to gently guide their focus toward specific chakras and help them more deeply connect with their inner energy centers.

The Seven Chakras:

- First Chakra: Root
- Second Chakra: Sacral
- Third Chakra: Solar Plexus
- Fourth Chakra: Heart
- Fifth Chakra: Throat
- Sixth Chakra: Third Eye
- Seventh Chakra: Crown

Clearing Energetic Blocks: One of the most common obstacles we face in life is an energetic block. These blocks manifest as barriers that prevent us from moving forward and achieving our full potential. While these blocks can appear in countless different forms, they all share one thing in common: they need to be cleared if we want to achieve success.

Fortunately, there is a simple and effective tool that can be used to clear these energetic blocks: the pendulum. A pendulum can be used to facilitate energetic cleansing. By pinpointing the areas where you feel stuck or blocked, you can identify the root cause of your issues and work to release them at their source. With time and practice, clearing your energetic blocks with a pendulum may help you move past old roadblocks and unlock your true potential.

There are hundreds of different ways that pendulums can be used, but at the core of their efficacy is the power of their vibrations. Pendulums help us to connect more deeply with our inner selves and the world around us, allowing us to access valuable insights and guidance at a deeper level than we can achieve on our own. Whether you're struggling with career decisions or trying to heal a particular issue in your life, pendulums can offer you helpful guidance and support at every step of the way.

DIFFERENT TYPES OF MATERIALS USED TO MAKE PENDULUM

There are many different types of materials that can be used to make pendulums, including crystals, wood, glass, and metals. The properties of each material determine the type of energy that the pendulum will conduct.

Crystals

Crystals are popular choices for making pendulums because they are thought to have special healing powers. Crystals generate energy at the molecular level and can help to align and balance our chakras and energy centers.

Additionally, crystal pigments are believed to react with our bodies to promote relaxation, improve concentration, relieve stress and anxiety, boost confidence, and combat negative emotions such as anger and depression. This suggests that using a crystal pendulum may be especially helpful for those who engage in meditation or other forms of personal reflection or introspection.

Here are some crystals and their specific purposes:

Rose Quartz: Rose quartz is an incredibly powerful stone that has long been revered for its ability to attract love, engage the soul, and foster deep connection. This beautiful stone is renowned for its vibrant hue and delicate rose-like texture, and it is known to help those seeking romance by infusing their lives with romantic vibes.

Additionally, rose quartz is believed to strengthen bonds of friendship, family unity, intimacy, and even platonic love, making it an excellent choice for those looking to deepen their existing relationships or discover new ones.

Clear Quartz: Clear quartz is a type of crystal that is prized for its energizing and cleansing properties. This mineral is known for its light, almost pure white color, which gives it a natural luminescence. Because clear quartz can absorb, amplify, and direct energy, it is often used in many different types of spiritual and energy work.

Whether used to promote healing and harmony or to enhance meditation and mindfulness, clear quartz is an effective tool in helping people to achieve their goals. When utilized correctly, this powerful crystal can help you achieve greater focus, clarity of mind, and increased vitality. Simply put, clear quartz can energize your body and spirit like nothing else!

Malachite: Malachite is a beautiful mineral that has been valued for its healing properties for thousands of years. This stone is known for its ability to promote emotional healing and boost confidence and courage. It has also been found to help alleviate feelings of anxiety and depression, making it useful for managing emotional stress. Furthermore, malachite has been shown to possess powerful anti-inflammatory properties, which can help speed up wound healing and reduce pain.

Lapis Lazuli: Lapis lazuli is a beautiful blue stone known for its deep metaphysical properties. Considered to be an ancient symbol of inner truth, lapis lazuli has long been used in meditations and spiritual practices as a way to help clear away negative energy and thoughts that obstruct mental clarity.

This powerful stone is also believed to enhance intuition, helping people tap into their inner wisdom and navigate the world with confidence. Whether you are looking to deepen your spiritual practice or simply find greater peace of mind, lapis lazuli can serve as an invaluable tool on your journey toward self-discovery.

Amethyst: Amethyst is a beautiful purple stone associated with healing and balance on both a physical and spiritual level. Known for its power to soothe and calm emotional turmoil, amethyst has long been used by healers to ease stress and anxiety.

Additionally, this gem is believed to help enhance meditation and psychic abilities, making it an ideal tool for those seeking deeper spiritual awareness. Whether you are seeking relief from emotional strain or simply want to enhance your psychic abilities, amethyst is an important stone that can help guide you along the path of personal growth and transformation.

Aventurine: Aventurine is a unique gemstone that is known for its properties of bringing good luck, promoting positivity and well-being, and spurring creativity. This powerful stone is believed to draw off negative energy and block electromagnetic pollution and radiation, making it a wonderful choice for anyone looking to boost their health or life satisfaction.

Additionally, thanks to its grounding nature and association with confidence and mental clarity, aventurine can help increase mental focus and clarity, enabling you to accomplish your goals with ease. Whether you're looking for a confidence boost or some extra energy to stay on top of your hectic schedule, aventurine is a perfect choice!

Carnelian: Carnelian is a type of stone that has been prized by ancient civilizations around the world for its beauty and ability to promote feelings of self-esteem and self-confidence. Known for its bright red hue, this gemstone exudes warmth and vitality, helping to foster feelings of inner strength and self-assurance.

In addition, carnelian is believed to aid in the flow of energy throughout the body, helping individuals feel more grounded and centered. Whether worn as jewelry or simply held in the hand, carnelian is a powerful tool for boosting one's sense of self-worth and encouraging deep personal growth.

Sodalite: Sodalite has long been prized for its calming and centering properties. This beautiful blue mineral is thought to be beneficial for anyone seeking stillness and focus, particularly in today's fast-paced world. In addition to its mental benefits, sodalite is also said to promote emotional well-being by encouraging harmony and balance within the body.

Some believe this quality can even help with mindfulness, as it directs focus toward the present moment instead of getting lost in stressful thoughts or worries about the future. Whether used as a meditation aid or simply enjoyed as a colorful addition to a room, sodalite is sure to bring welcome peace and tranquility into any home or workplace.

Amazonite: Amazonite is a beautiful stone with many unique properties that make it ideal for those who are struggling with anger or stress. For example, the calming effect of amazonite can help to reduce feelings of hostility or irritability, enabling the user to stay focused and grounded even in challenging situations.

Additionally, by enhancing tranquility and putting the user at ease, amazonite helps to cultivate stability and sweetness in difficult periods. Furthermore, amazonite also works on an energetic level, drawing out negative patterns in our behavior so that we can become more aware of them and hopefully choose to change them.

Tiger Eye: Tiger eye is a gemstone known for its ability to help support positive transformation and energy. With its distinctive golden-brown color, the tiger eye is believed to possess many powerful properties. It is thought to have strong grounding qualities that can promote emotional balance and help to alleviate worry and fear.

Additionally, the tiger eye is believed to be an energizing stone that can enhance creativity, motivation, and determination. Thus, this unique gemstone has become a popular tool in practices such as crystal healing and energy work, helping people to harness the power of natural energies for the betterment of themselves and their surroundings.

Fluorite: The mineral fluorite is well-known for the exceptional clarity it has as well as its high refractive index. As a result of this, it has developed into a well-liked option for usage in the production of lenses and windows. It is believed that fluorite's capabilities as a natural amplifier enable it to assist individuals in improving the quality of their decision-making processes by increasing the clarity and concentration of their thinking.

Because of this, it is an excellent option for people who want to increase their ability to solve problems or refine their intuition, since it enables them to see patterns and subtle indications that could otherwise go overlooked. If you are looking to advance your career or simply want to boost your overall productivity, fluorite can be an extremely useful tool for enhancing your mental acuity and sharpening your decision-making abilities. This is true whether you are looking to advance your career or simply want to boost your overall productivity.

Rhodonite: Rhodonite is a stunning gemstone that is frequently connected with feelings of love, including self-love. This one-of-a-kind stone is distinguished by the dark red coloration and striking striations that it possesses. Rhodonite may give the impression that it is a solid stone; nevertheless, it is highly porous, which enables it to take in certain energies from its surrounding environment.

Because of this feature of rhodonite, having the stone in your bedroom or in the location where you meditate can facilitate a deeper connection to sentiments of love and compassion, both for yourself and other people. In addition, relaxing energies might assist you in feeling more connected to your actual nature and the sense of purpose that you have in your life.

Labradorite: Labradorite is a kind of gemstone that is famous for its iridescent sheen and shimmering look. The mineral was first discovered in the Canadian province of Labrador, from whence it gets its name. However, it has since been discovered in several other places, including Finland and Madagascar. This particular stone is well-known for possessing several beneficial attributes, one of which is the capacity to bestow bravery, strength, and power in the face of hardship.

In addition to this, it is a useful strategy for controlling one's emotions and maintaining composure in high-stress situations. Labradorite is a strong gem that can assist enhance our lives in a variety of significant ways. It is known for its ability to boost one's energy levels and to have a relaxing influence on the mind.

This multipurpose stone always has something to give, whether we are seeking empowerment in challenging circumstances or looking for a means to channel tension and worry into productive action.

Fancy Jasper: It is well-known that the semi-precious stone known as Fancy Jasper has the power to improve one's concentration and clarity. This stunning stone has a vivid and brilliant look, which distinguishes it from the innumerable other stones that can be found across the world.

Fancy jasper is frequently utilized in meditation, crystal healing, and the balancing of chakras due to the energy-enhancing capabilities that it possesses. Fancy jasper not only helps us maintain our attention and focus, but it also fosters clear decision-making and stimulates rapid thinking in difficult situations.

Hematite: One of the most powerful tools for removing bad energy from your mind, body, and soul is the hematite crystal. Hematite is also known as iron pyrite. Hematite, which is famous for its extraordinary capacity to absorb energy, may help you achieve maximum development and healing by clearing your aura of any obstacles that may be standing in the way of your progress. Hematite gives a significant boost to one's mental and physical well-being, whether it is through the alleviation of stress or the promotion of the discovery of novel chances.

Aventurine: It has been believed for a very long time that individuals who wear aventurine would be blessed with good fortune and pleasant energy. Aventurine is a gorgeous stone that can be used in a variety of different ways. This crystal is most commonly seen in brilliant green color, although it also occurs in orange, yellow, brown, blue, and red hues. Its green tint is what gives it its name.

Aventurine is a stone that is frequently linked to positive attributes like prosperity, success in one's job, and general happiness and health. This stone's energizing qualities and luxurious feel make it an excellent tool for bolstering self-assurance and fostering contentment, even amid challenging circumstances.

Pyrite: Pyrite is a versatile mineral that has been held in high esteem for a long time as an influential representation of success and wealth. This metallic stone has been used in talismans, amulets, and several other types of magical implements for hundreds of years, earning it the nickname "fool's gold" due to its unusual look and yellowish tone.

Pyrite has, throughout history, been associated with concepts relating to plenty and good fortune. It has the potential to assist in motivating us toward the accomplishment of our goals while also offering powerful energy support. This magnificent stone is likely to stimulate feelings of optimism, hope, and success regardless of whether you use pyrite crystals in your house or take them with you when you go out and about.

Blue Onyx: Onyx is a strong stone that has long been connected with bravery and protection. Blue Onyx is one of the most well-known varieties. This mineral may be found in many different parts of the world, and it is easily distinguished from other types of stones due to its characteristic pale blue tint.

It is claimed that Blue Onyx includes a range of nutrients and minerals that have beneficial benefits on the body, such as strengthening one's bravery and sense of willpower. This is in addition to the fact that Blue Onyx has a powerful look. Because of this, it is an excellent option for anyone who wants to lift their spirits or protect themselves from the negative influences they encounter in their day-to-day life.

However, perhaps most crucially, Blue Onyx is recognized for its extraordinary capacity to absorb negative energies and then release them back into the environment as positive energy. This is perhaps the most essential characteristic of Blue Onyx. This potent mineral can be of assistance to you on your path to obtaining inner tranquility and happiness, whether you are currently dealing with a challenging circumstance or you simply desire a higher level of harmony in your life.

Wood

Pendulums are also frequently crafted from wood, which is another material that is employed. Because wood is a representation of nature, it has the power to make us feel more connected to the natural world around us and to inspire us to take things more slowly and spend more time outside. In addition, we can promote a feeling of stability and grounding by drawing on the earth's energy that is contained inside the wood. This may be useful for individuals who are going through challenging times or who are coping with emotional issues.

Pendulums made of wood are a very useful and trustworthy instrument for divination and getting answers. Wooden pendulums, on the other hand, can only react to the person who is holding them, in contrast to crystal pendulums, which are typically connected with healing in addition to providing answers. Because of this, they are an excellent option for people who are looking for particular answers or directions, as the user can restrict the amount of energy that builds up between them and their pendulum.

In addition, in comparison to other forms of pendulums, wooden pendulums have several benefits to offer. Because they are constructed out of wood, they are often more durable than items manufactured from other materials and are less likely to become damaged or broken. Wood is also said to have a soothing impact on its users, making it an excellent option for people who favor a more grounded approach when looking for guidance or direction in their life.

Glass

Glass is a good medium for energy work because of its smooth surface, which helps to concentrate and magnify healing vibrations and makes it a responsive medium. Glass, on the other hand, possesses a distinctive capacity to store and channel energy, which makes it an excellent choice as a material for the fabrication of resonant healing implements.

In addition, because glass is virtually inert, the usage of these pendulums is entirely risk-free, and it is appropriate for practitioners of any level of expertise to employ them. Glass is an excellent option for those who are prone to changing their minds about the treatment techniques they want to pursue since it is easier to clean and maintain than other materials.

Metals

Because they are associated with the element of Earth, metals are also frequently utilized in the production of pendulums. A lot of people think that if we wear a piece of jewelry made of metal, it will help us connect with the energies of the earth in a deeper way, which will in turn boost our capacity to cure ourselves.

Copper, for instance, is regarded to be very good for enhancing blood flow and strengthening the immune system. [Citation needed] [Citation needed] In the meanwhile, it is believed that silver can help alleviate pain and bring inflammation in the body under control. On the other side, gold is said to exude a good aura and is connected with vigor.

Your one-of-a-kind requirements and personal preferences will determine the kind of material that is utilized to make a pendulum. Nevertheless, regardless of the material, using a pendulum can prove to be an efficient method for gaining access to our inner wisdom and fostering profound healing on both the physical and emotional levels.

THE DIFFERENT SHAPES OF PENDULUM

There are many different shapes and designs for pendulums, each of which may offer its unique benefits. Some of the most popular options include:

Circular pendulums: These pendulums typically feature a small weight at the end of a chain or cord. They are often favored by beginners because they are easy to hold and use. At the same time, circular pendulums are also a great choice for experienced practitioners who want to explore more advanced techniques.

Rectangular Pendulums: Rectangular pendulums are said to be good for general healing, as they promote balance and harmony in the body. They are also said to help clear negative energy from the aura.

Cone Pendulums: Cone pendulums are used to explore the spiritual realm. Known for their ability to stimulate the chakras and promote spiritual growth, cone pendulums are believed to help access hidden knowledge, explore different planes of consciousness, and better understand the subconscious mind.

Pyramid Pendulums: Pyramid pendulums are said to be good for focus and concentration, as well as for amplifying the energies of other crystals. They are also said to help manifest one's desires and goals.

Sphere Pendulums: Sphere pendulums are said to be good for promoting peace and tranquility, as well as for easing stress and anxiety. They are also said to help achieve clarity of thought and enhance psychic abilities.

Egg Pendulums: Egg pendulums are said to be good for fertility and new beginnings, as well as for promoting creativity and imagination. They are also said to help ward off negative energy and attract positive energy.

Disc Pendulums: Disc pendulums are said to be good for protection and grounding, as well as for deflecting negative energy. They are also said to help balance the chakras and align the subtle bodies.

Column Pendulums: Column pendulums are said to be good for strength and stability, as well as for promoting mental clarity and aiding in decision-making. They are also said to help access past lives and understand karmic patterns.

Oval Pendulums: Oval pendulums are said to be good for emotional healing, as they help to release blocked emotions and promote self-love. They are also said to help attract abundance and prosperity.

<u>**Chambered Pendulums:**</u> Chambered pendulums are a special kind of pendulum that can have anywhere from one to many chambers inside of it. Crystal practitioners and energy workers will find these chambers to be an extremely useful tool because they may be utilized to build a diverse range of connections and focal places.

You may, for instance, fill the chamber with essential oils or crystal chips to aid facilitate healing, eliminate energetic blocks, or materialize the things you want in your life. When working with the energies of the cosmos, chambered pendulums are meant to assist you in maintaining your sense of balance and concentration, which is perhaps the most significant benefit.

The use of a pendulum can be an effective method for gaining access to one's inner knowledge and fostering profound healing on several levels, including the physical, the emotional, and the mental. It doesn't matter if you're just getting started with dowsing or if you've been doing it for years; the form and type of pendulum that you use should be tailored to your needs.

HOW TO SHOP FOR A PENDULUM?

When shopping for a pendulum, it is important to keep a few important considerations in mind. When you hold the pendulum, it is of the utmost importance that it be familiar and easy to do so; this should be your first and primary concern. The availability of a diverse range of pendulums from a variety of online stores, such as Etsy, appeals to a large number of consumers and encourages them to purchase online.

Alternately, if you have previous experience creating things yourself, you might want to think about attempting to construct your pendulum out of materials that feel natural to you. This is an option to explore if you have previous experience producing things. In the end, it is essential to do some research on the many varieties of pendulums available so that you may select one that satisfies both your tastes and your requirements.

5-STEP GUIDE TO GET STARTED IN USING A PENDULUM

A pendulum is an excellent instrument for practicing divination and gaining new insights. Additionally, even novices will have no trouble figuring out how to utilize it. To be able to concentrate, all you want is a pendulum and some peace. You may start utilizing a pendulum to find answers to your concerns in a matter of just a few straightforward steps.

Step One: Arm yourself with basic knowledge and important safety precautions

It is important to arm yourself with some important rules and safety precautions before beginning the usage of a pendulum since this will allow you to get started. The first thing you should do is ensure that you have sufficient knowledge of how to use a pendulum. This involves having a fundamental grasp of the subject, such as how the swing of a pendulum might be utilized for divination.

You must acquaint yourself with typical safety measures before beginning a session. For example, while you are using your pendulum, you should handle it with care, and you should practice proper grounding before you begin. You will put yourself in a position to be successful while utilizing your pendulum if you prepare yourself by equipping yourself with this fundamental information and following suitable safety precautions.

Step Two: Pick your pendulum

The first thing to do while working with a pendulum is to select the pendulum that you will use. When it comes to choosing this choice, there are a lot of different aspects to think about, including the material and the shape of the pendulum itself. Depending on your own choice and the kinds of materials that have a spiritual resonance for you, some of the most common possibilities are crystals, wood, or metal.

In addition, there are additional considerations that may come into play, such as the size and weight of the pendulum. It is essential to choose a pendulum that will fit comfortably in your palm and provide sufficient stability for accurate readings. In the last section, we discussed the many varieties of pendulums, including their crystals, materials, and forms. When selecting a pendulum, you should also think about the length of the string, whether or not it is weighted, and whether or not it has any other attachments, such as crystals or religious symbols.

In the end, choosing a pendulum is a highly personal process that should be done cautiously and attentively to achieve the best results. Consequently, set aside a portion of your busy schedule to investigate the myriad of available choices and zero in on the one that resonates most strongly with you.

Step Three: Calibrate your pendulum

After you've decided which pendulum to use, the next thing you'll need to do is locate a peaceful and quiet place where you can hone your talents via practice and experimentation. This may be an office you have in your house, a private nook in one of your bedrooms, or even a spot outside, such as your yard or garden. Find a location that lets you unwind and concentrate on your job without any interruptions from the outside world, regardless of where you choose to put in your practice time.

Take several deep breaths, find a comfortable seat, and make sure your back is straight. This will help you get centered. You should be holding your pendulum in your dominant hand, which is the one you write with. At the same time, your arm should be relaxed by resting your elbow on a table or other surface in front of you. After taking one more calm, deep breath, exhale completely and then concentrate entirely on the movement of the pendulum. Swing it back and forth slowly so that your body can establish a connection with the tool. Doing so will make it simpler for you to get new ideas in the future.

At this point, you might wish to consider calibrating your pendulum with some fundamental recommendations regarding its use. To begin, make sure your pendulum is motionless as you ask it what "yes" means. Pay special attention to the path the pendulum takes as it swings; does it move in a vertical or horizontal plane, or does it move in a circular pattern? You should have no trouble recognizing this movement as a sign that the response is yes. It should be quite obvious to you.

After you have determined that the response "yes" possesses its unique motion, you can then continue with the process of calibrating the pendulum by asking it a question to which you already know the answer. Questions such as "Is my name John?" or "Am I 25 years old?" are appropriate places to begin, since they should offer you rapid feedback that you can use to calibrate your pendulum. These are also acceptable beginning points.

Once you have mastered the calibration procedure, which will take some time and experience, you will be able to swiftly discover the answers to any questions by just holding your pendulum in front of you and reading the motion of its swing. Now that you are equipped with this information, you may start making use of your pendulum to get insights into the spiritual realm and to perform healing sessions for both yourself and other people.

Step Four: Implement your purpose

Implementing your purpose is the fourth step in the process. The pendulum is a very potent instrument that may be used for a variety of purposes, including gaining insight into your energy centers, checking the energy of other people, clearing and balancing your chakras, and attracting a particular objective.

This multifaceted instrument of divination may also be used to discover misplaced items or energies that are blocking your flow, making it a very useful all-around tool. The pendulum's straightforward construction and user-friendly functioning make it possible for you to quickly and easily access the latent capabilities of your energy body, enhancing your level of awareness and bringing greater inner harmony into your life.

<u>Gain insight into your energy centers:</u> Hold your pendulum over one of your energy centers, such as your heart chakra or third eye, and ask it to reveal the status of that particular center. To get started, hold your pendulum over one of your energy centers. If the pendulum is moving at all, even a little, this is a sign that there are some obstructions in the region you are examining. You will be able to work on clearing any blockages and balancing your energy centers from this vantage point, which will allow you to experience better harmony, clarity, and calm in your day-to-day existence.

<u>Check the energy of others:</u> A further popular application for the pendulum is to gauge the energy of those in the vicinity of the user. To accomplish this, just hold it over the body of the person you wish to examine (or over the specific area of their body where you have reason to believe there may be problems) and ask it to display the information you require. Pay attention to how the pendulum swings since this will reveal whether or not the energy of that individual is in line or whether any obstacles are limiting their progress.

<u>Clear and balance your chakras:</u> Clearing and balancing your chakras may also be accomplished efficiently by making use of a pendulum. You should start by holding the pendulum over each of your seven energy centers and asking what needs to be done to remove any blockages or bring greater flow and balance into that region.

You should do this while asking the pendulum to show you what needs to be done. This might entail having an intuitive understanding of which crystal is most suited for a specific chakra, envisioning the state of equilibrium that is sought, or just taking a few deep breaths to assist bring calm and focus into your energy field.

<u>Attract a specific goal:</u> The pendulum is a fantastic tool to use if you want to improve your chances of achieving a certain objective or achieving the desired result in your life. Simply hold it over your body and ask it to teach you how you can become in alignment with the objective that you have set for yourself. This might entail employing techniques like affirmations and visualizations to assist you in achieving the result you want, or it could mean doing the work that needs to be done to get closer to your objective.

<u>Locate lost objects:</u> It is essential to start by holding the pendulum in your hands before attempting to utilize it as a tool for finding lost items while using a pendulum. Put your attention squarely on the thing you're trying to find, and see it as vividly as you can in your mind. The next step is to inquire as to the location of the item in question by posing inquiries such as, "Is it in my bedroom?" Pay great attention to the pendulum while you carry out this procedure and note any movements or shifts that it undergoes. Your response, whether it be yes or no, may then be determined based on the information provided.

<u>Locate energies that are stuck in your flow:</u> Start by holding the pendulum over a particular area of your body or energy field where you have a hunch there may be blockages. This is the first step in using a pendulum to discover energies that are trapped in your flow.

Pendulums are available at most metaphysical supply stores. Ask it to show you what is holding you back and how you can remove those blockages of energy so that you can go forward. This might include imagining certain energy traveling through your body, or it could simply involve taking some deep breaths to assist in releasing any energies that have been trapped.

A pendulum is a powerful tool that, despite its straightforward construction and straightforward operation, can be used to do a wide variety of things, including discovering your latent potential, gaining insight into your energy centers, checking the energy of others, clearing and balancing your chakras, and attracting a particular goal.

The use of a pendulum, whether you are new to energy work and healing or have years of expertise under your belt, may assist you in gaining better clarity and insight into your inner self as well as those around you.

Step Five: Take care of your pendulum

It is essential to approach your pendulum with the utmost care and deference if you want to get the most out of it. Always address the pendulum with kindness, using a relaxed and kind tone of voice, and speaking softly to ensure that it functions properly.

In addition, it is essential to avoid forcing or pushing your pendulum to obtain answers, as doing so might result in inaccurate readings. You may guarantee that the information you obtain from your divinatory tool, such as a pendulum, is as accurate and useful as possible by paying attention to these pointers and following the correct procedures for dealing with your pendulum.

Conclusion

The ability to harness the transformational potential of energy is essential in the process of bringing a goal into physical manifestation. Using a pendulum as a means to do this is one approach that may be used. A pendulum is a little device that is suspended by a thread or chain. By swinging the pendulum back and forth, one can tap into the forces of energy that are there to facilitate healing on both the physical and spiritual levels.

This kind of instrument has the potential to provide a multitude of advantages. To begin, one can change particular energy frequencies according to their needs by adjusting the direction in which they hold and move the pendulum as well as the speed at which they do so and the amount of intensity with which they do so.

Second, by using a pendulum, one may determine whether or not there are imbalances in one's general energy system, which may be the cause of unfavorable symptoms in one's day-to-day life. If we can detect these imbalances at an early stage, we will have more time to work toward resolving them before they create any long-term damage.

And lastly, during therapy sessions with the pendulum, we may strengthen our natural healing energies so that we feel more energetic, balanced, and entire all around by concentrating on certain locations or target frequencies. This is done by focusing on specific areas or target frequencies.

In conclusion, it is abundantly obvious that making use of a pendulum is an efficient approach to accessing the transforming potential of energy that is inside each of us to facilitate the healing of the mind and the body. Utilizing this tool will help you restore your equilibrium and assist you toward reaching your objectives and creating good changes in your life, regardless of whether you are struggling with medical issues or emotional challenges such as stress or despair.

So, the next time you find yourself in a rut or lacking inspiration on how to go forward with your objectives here's one approach to consider: get moving! Energy therapies are just around the corner with the assistance of the curative qualities of a good old-fashioned pendulum.

FAQ

1. What is a pendulum?

A pendulum is a weight, typically made of metal or stone, that is attached to a cord or chain. Pendulums are used for divination, which is a form of fortune telling that involves using an object to answer questions or predict the future.

2. How does a pendulum work?

Pendulums work by harnessing the power of the subconscious mind. When a question is asked, the subconscious mind will provide an answer by moving the pendulum in a certain direction.

3. What are the different types of pendulums?

There are many different types of pendulums, each with its unique properties. Some of the most popular types of pendulums include crystal pendulums, metal pendulums, and wood pendulums.

4. How do I choose a pendulum?

The type of pendulum you choose should be based on your personal preferences and needs. If you are looking for a general-purpose pendulum, then a crystal or metal pendulum would be a good choice. If you are looking for a specific type of reading, then you may want to choose a pendulum that is made from a material that corresponds to that reading (e.g., using a wood pendulum for an earth reading).

5. How do I use a pendulum?

To use a pendulum for divination, you will need to first calibrate it to your energy field. This can be done by holding the pendulum in your dominant hand and asking it to show you your "yes" response. Once the pendulum has been calibrated, you can ask it any yes or no question that you desire. The answer will be indicated by the direction in which the pendulum swings (e.g., clockwise for yes, counterclockwise for no).

6. What are some tips for using a pendulum?

Here are some tips for using a pendulum:

- Relax your mind and body before beginning your reading. This will help to ensure that your readings are accurate.
- Be clear and concise when asking questions. The more specific your question is, the more accurate your reading will be.
- Trust your intuition when interpreting the answers given by your pendulum. Sometimes the answer may not make logical sense, but if it feels right then it probably is!

- Keep track of your readings so that you can look back on them later and see how they have unfolded over time.

7. What are some common misconceptions about pendulums?

One common misconception about Pendulums is that they can be used to control other people or objects through magical means. Another misconception is that Pendulums can only give yes or no answers to questions asked of them when this is not always true as sometimes more complicated answers present themselves through swing patterns or movement speeds. Additionally, some people think that anyone can use a Pendulum without any training when in reality it does take some practice to get used to both interpretations of the signals given as well as avoid bias in readings due to personal beliefs.

8. Can anyone learn how to use a pendulum?

Yes! While it may take some time and practice to get comfortable with both using and interpreting Pendulum readings, with patience and an open mind almost anyone can learn this skill. It's important to remember however that not everyone will experience success with Pendulum readings - just as some people don't believe in their accuracy - so if at first, you don't feel like you're getting anywhere, don't get discouraged!

9. Do I need any special equipment to use a pendulum?

No! All you need to start using Pendulums for divination purposes is one weight - often made from metal, stone, glass, wood, or even plastic - which hangs from either a cord or chain. You may also want something to act as a base upon which to rest your Pendulum while working such as an upturned glass, small bowl, plate, or even just a clean flat surface. However, many people believe that certain materials can add additional power or meaning readings so feel free to experiment until you find what works best for you!

10. Are there any dangers associated with using pendulums?

While there is no concrete evidence that using pendulums poses any real danger beyond potentially inaccurate readings if not used correctly, some people nevertheless worry about becoming possessed by evil spirits or entities when working with Divination tools like this. If this concern resonates with you then it might be best to avoid using it.

References

Estrada, J. (2021, August 5). If you're indecisive, you need a pendulum in your mystical tool kit. Cosmopolitan. https://www.cosmopolitan.com/lifestyle/a37234650/how-to-use-a-pendulum/.

Houston, D. (2019, May 18). How to use a pendulum – the complete guide. CrystalsandJewelry.Com. https://meanings.crystalsandjewelry.com/pendulum/.

How to use a pendulum. (n.d.). Learn Religions. Retrieved November 4, 2022, from https://www.learnreligions.com/use-a-pendulum-1725780.

Pendulum Therapy: How to use a Pendulum for balancing the body energy. (n.d.). The Times of India. Retrieved November 4, 2022, from https://timesofindia.indiatimes.com/life-style/health-fitness/de-stress/pendulum-therapy-how-to-use-a-pendulum-for-balancing-the-body-energy/articleshow/70789040.cms.

Pendulum dowsing – an introduction to using a pendulum. (n.d.). Holistic Shop. Retrieved November 4, 2022, from https://www.holisticshop.co.uk/articles/guide-pendulum-dowsing.

Rhodonite: Meaning, healing properties and powers. (n.d.). Retrieved November 4, 2022, from https://www.mycrystals.com/meaning/rhodonite-meaning-healing-properties-and-powers.

The ultimate pendulum guide. (n.d.). My Little Magic Shop. Retrieved November 4, 2022, from https://mylittlemagicshop.com/blogs/magical-words/the-ultimate-pendulum-guide.